HEALING HERBS FOR SOBRIETY: 25 NATURAL REMEDIES TO SUPPORT YOUR RECOVERY

Deidra Marie

INTRODUCTION

Embarking on the journey to sobriety is both challenging and rewarding. It is a path that requires strength, resilience, and a willingness to embrace change. As someone who has walked this path, I can attest to the transformative power of this journey. One of the most significant aspects of my healing process has been the use of herbs. These natural allies have supported me in detoxifying my body, calming my mind, and bringing my entire being into balance. This book aims to share the knowledge and wisdom I've gained about using herbs to support sobriety.

The journey to sobriety is deeply personal, and everyone's path is unique. For me, discovering the world of herbalism was a turning point. After years of living with alcohol dependence, I found solace and healing in the simple yet profound act of incorporating herbs into my daily routine. Herbs like dandelion, milk thistle, and burdock root helped to detoxify my body, cleansing it from the toxins accumulated over years of alcohol and tobacco use. Nervine herbs like chamomile, lemon balm, and skullcap provided much-needed relief from anxiety and stress, which often accompany the early stages of sobriety.

In addition to detoxifying and calming herbs, I discovered a new group of herbs I was unfamiliar with, adaptogens. These herbs, including ashwagandha, holy basil, and ginseng, helped bring my body into homeostasis, supporting my overall health and well being. By incorporating these herbs into my daily routine, I was able to find a sense of balance and stability that had eluded me for what now seems like my entire life. I call this group of herbs "my energetic coat of armor".

In this book, you will find information on these herbs that can support your sobriety journey. Each chapter is dedicated to a specific category of herbs, including detoxifying herbs, nervine herbs, and adaptogens. You will learn about the benefits of each herb, how to use them, and different preparation methods. Whether you prefer herbal teas, tinctures, capsules, or herb-infused oils, this book provides practical guidance on incorporating these natural remedies into your daily life.

One of the most rewarding aspects of my journey has been growing and making my own herbal remedies. Inspired by the profound impact herbs had on my healing, I decided to take herbalism courses and create a botanical beverage garden. Today, I cultivate 20 different herbs, depending on the season, and make teas, tinctures and other preparations with fresh herbs straight from the garden. This daily ritual has become a cornerstone of my sobriety, grounding and healing me in ways I could not have imagined.

The 25 herbal recipes are designed to support your recovery. From detoxifying teas to calming tinctures and soothing salves, these herbs and preparations are easy to locate for purchase or simple to prepare and incorporate into your daily routine. My hope is that these recipes will inspire you to explore the world of herbs and discover their incredible benefits for yourself.

Sobriety is a journey, not a destination. It requires ongoing commitment and self-care. By embracing the healing power of herbs, you can support your body, mind, and spirit in the most holistic way possible. May this book serve as a guide and inspiration on your path to recovery.

Anaïs Nin

"And the day came when the risk to remain tight in a bud was more painful than the risk it took to blossom."

HERBAL USE THROUGH HISTORY

Herbal medicine, also known as herbalism or phytotherapy, is the practice of using plants and plant extracts for medicinal purposes. This ancient practice dates back thousands of years and has been integral to the healing traditions of many cultures worldwide.

Ancient Civilizations

- **Egypt:** Ancient Egyptians documented their use of herbs on papyrus scrolls, such as the Ebers Papyrus, which lists over 850 plant medicines. Herbs like garlic, juniper, and aloe vera were commonly used.
- **China:** Traditional Chinese Medicine (TCM) has a rich history of herbal use, with texts like the "Shennong Ben Cao Jing" detailing the medicinal properties of hundreds of herbs. TCM focuses on balancing the body's energy, or Qi, using herbs like ginseng and licorice root.
- **India:** Ayurveda, the traditional medicine system of India, has used herbs for thousands of years. Ayurvedic texts like the "Charaka Samhita" describe the medicinal use of plants such as turmeric, ashwagandha, and holy basil to promote balance in the body's doshas.

Indigenous Cultures

- Indigenous peoples around the world have used local plants for healing. Native American tribes, for example, used herbs like echinacea and willow bark for their medicinal properties. These practices are often passed down through generations and are deeply intertwined with cultural traditions and spiritual beliefs.

Medieval Europe

- In medieval Europe, monasteries were centers of herbal knowledge. Monks cultivated medicinal gardens and transcribed ancient texts, preserving herbal knowledge through the Dark Ages. The "Physica" by Hildegard of Bingen and the "Herbarium" by Apuleius Platonicus are notable works from this period.

Modern Herbalism

- Today, herbalism is recognized as a complementary and alternative medicine. With a resurgence of interest in natural and holistic health, many people turn to herbs for their therapeutic benefits. Modern herbalists combine traditional knowledge with scientific research to offer safe and effective herbal remedies.

Methods Of Incorporating Herbs Into Daily Life

Herbal Teas

- Herbal teas, or tisanes, are made by steeping herbs in hot water. This method is simple and allows for easy absorption of the herb's beneficial compounds. Teas can be made from leaves, flowers, roots, or seeds, and can be enjoyed hot or cold.

Tinctures

- Tinctures are concentrated herbal extracts made

by soaking herbs in a solvent, traditionally alcohol. However, for those avoiding alcohol, apple cider vinegar or glycerin can be used as a menstruum. Tinctures are potent and have a long shelf life. They are typically taken in small doses using a dropper.

Capsules and Tablets

- Herbs can be dried, ground into powder, and encapsulated for easy consumption. This method is convenient for those who prefer not to taste the herbs directly. Capsules and tablets provide a consistent dosage and are readily available at health food stores or can be made at home.

Herb-Infused Oils

- Infusing herbs in oil extracts their fat-soluble compounds, which can be used for culinary or topical applications. Herbal oils can be used in cooking, as salad dressings, or for massage and skincare. Commonly used oils include olive oil, coconut oil, and jojoba oil.

Salves and Balms

- Salves and balms are made by combining herb-infused oils with beeswax or another solidifying agent. These are used topically to heal and soothe the skin. They are particularly effective for treating cuts, burns, and other skin conditions.

Hydrosols

- Hydrosols are the aromatic water produced during the steam distillation of plants. They contain the water-soluble compounds of the plant and are used as facial toners, room sprays, or in culinary applications. Hydrosols are gentler than essential oils and can be used directly on the skin.

Essential Oils

- Essential oils are highly concentrated plant extracts obtained through steam distillation or cold pressing. They are used in aromatherapy, skincare, and as natural remedies for various ailments. Due to their potency, essential oils should be used with caution and often need to be diluted before application.

Essential Considerations For Herbal Use

Safety and Precautions

- While herbs are natural, they are also powerful and should be used with care. It's essential to consult with a healthcare provider before starting any herbal regimen, especially if you are pregnant, breastfeeding, or taking other medications. Be aware of potential allergies and interactions with other herbs and medications.

Quality and Sourcing

- The effectiveness of herbal remedies depends on the quality of the herbs used. It's crucial to source herbs from reputable suppliers who use sustainable and organic farming practices. Freshness is also vital, as dried herbs can lose potency over time.

Sustainability

- Ethical harvesting and sustainable practices are essential in herbalism. Overharvesting can deplete wild plant populations and harm ecosystems. Whenever possible, use cultivated herbs or support companies that practice sustainable wildcrafting.

By understanding the rich history of herbal medicine, the various methods of incorporating herbs into your daily life, and the importance of safety and sustainability, you can harness the power of nature to support your sobriety journey. May this knowledge empower you to explore the world of herbs and discover their incredible benefits for yourself.

Lao Tzu

"The journey of a thousand miles begins with one step."

PREFACE

The journey to sobriety is a deeply personal and transformative one. It requires strength, resilience, and a great deal of support. My own path to sobriety has been profoundly influenced by the healing power of herbs. This book is a culmination of my experiences and the knowledge I've gained along the way. It is my hope that these natural remedies will offer you the support and healing they have provided me.

Each chapter of this book is designed to guide you through the process of using herbs to support your recovery. From detoxifying your body to calming your mind and balancing your overall health, these herbs are nature's gift to us. You will find 25 herbal recipes that are simple to prepare and incorporate into your daily routine.

May this book serve as a source of inspiration and practical guidance on your journey in sobriety.

Haruki Murakami

"And once the storm is over, you won't remember how you made it through, how you managed to survive. You won't even be sure whether the storm is really over. But one thing is certain. When you come out of the storm, you won't be the same person who walked in."

CHAPTER 1: MY HERBAL JOURNEY

Although herbs have been a part of my life for many years, it wasn't until I embarked on my journey to sobriety that I truly discovered their incredible potential. I turned to my herbal allies during the process of removing alcohol because I knew they would help me detox my body, reduce my anxiety and overwhelm, and balance my mood swings and cravings. In this way, herbs can be trusted companions, offering unwavering support when needed the most.

The journey began with something as simple as herbal teas. I reached for calming herbs like chamomile, skullcap and lemon balm, knowing they would soothe my anxious mind and help me sleep better. The warmth of the tea, the gentle aroma, and the sense of peace they brought me were profound. It felt like a comforting hug in a cup, a small but significant step towards healing. This reignited my passion for herbalism and motivated me to explore further.

As I delved deeper, I began experimenting with various herbs and preparations. Detoxifying herbs like dandelion and milk thistle played a crucial role in cleansing my body from the toxins accumulated over years of alcohol use and cigarettes. These herbs didn't just improve my physical health; they revitalized my spirit, giving me the energy and clarity I had been longing for.

Four years ago, my journey took a significant turn. Inspired by the profound impact herbs had on my life, I decided to deepen my knowledge and enrolled in formal herbalism courses. These courses were eye-opening. They revealed the intricate science behind the plants' medicinal properties and taught me various methods of preparing and using them. I learned to make tinctures, salves, and herb-infused oils, and I discovered a deep appreciation for the art and science of herbal remedies.

Around this time, I also started my own botanical beverage garden. Growing my own herbs felt like a natural progression, allowing me to ensure the highest quality and potency of the plants I used. My garden, which now boasts around 20 different herbs depending on the season, became my sanctuary. The act of nurturing these plants, harvesting them at their peak, and creating remedies from fresh herbs straight from the garden became a daily ritual that grounded me in ways I had never experienced before.

Herbalism opened up a new world of calm that I had not known previously. The process of growing and making herbal remedies helped me slow down tremendously. It connected me to nature in a profound way and provided a sense of fulfillment and purpose. Each step, from planting the seeds to sipping a freshly brewed tea, became a mindful practice that brought me peace and joy.

Herbalism has transformed my life in ways I could not have imagined. It provided me with the tools to support my sobriety, manage my stress, and enhance my overall health. More importantly, it gave me a sense of purpose and fulfillment. Through my journey, I have become an advocate for the healing power of herbs and am passionate about sharing this knowledge with others.

I hope that by sharing my story and the wisdom I have gained, I can inspire others to explore the world of herbs and discover their incredible benefits. Whether you are on a journey to sobriety or simply seeking natural ways to enhance your well-being, I encourage you to embrace the healing power of herbs. They have the potential to transform your life, just as they have transformed mine.

Ralph Waldo Emerson

"What lies behind us and what lies before us are tiny matters compared to what lies within us."

DAILY ROUTINE AND LIFESTYLE EVALUATION

This assessment aims to provide a clear picture of your current daily habits and routines, helping you identify the best ways to integrate herbal remedies into your lifestyle. Understanding your routine can help ensure that the incorporation of herbs is seamless and sustainable.

Questions

1. **Current Herbal Use**
   - How often do you currently consume herbal teas or other herbal products?
     - Daily
     - Several times a week
     - Occasionally
     - Never

2. **Self-Care Routine**
   - Do you have a set routine for self-care?
     - Yes, every morning
     - Yes, every evening
     - Yes, both morning and evening
     - No, it varies

- No, I don't have a set routine
- If you have a self-care routine, please describe it briefly.
  - What activities do you include (e.g., meditation, exercise, skincare)?
  - How long do you usually take?

3. **Time Management**
- How much time can you dedicate to preparing and using herbal remedies each day?
  - Less than 10 minutes
  - 10-20 minutes
  - 20-30 minutes
  - More than 30 minutes

4. **Preferred Methods of Consumption**
- What are your preferred methods for consuming herbs? (Select all that apply)
  - Herbal teas
  - Capsules or tablets
  - Tinctures
  - Herb-infused oils
  - Topical applications (e.g., salves, balms)
  - Aromatherapy (e.g., essential oils, hydrosols)

5. **Meal Patterns**
- How many meals do you eat per day?
  - 1-2
  - 3
  - 4 or more
- Do you include any herbal ingredients in your meals? If yes, which ones?

6. **Hydration Habits**
- How much water do you drink daily?
  - Less than 4 cups
  - 4-6 cups
  - 6-8 cups
  - More than 8 cups
- Do you drink any herbal beverages besides water? If yes, which ones?

7. **Sleep Patterns**
- How many hours of sleep do you get on average per night?
  - Less than 5 hours
  - 5-6 hours
  - 6-7 hours
  - 7-8 hours
  - More than 8 hours
- Do you have any bedtime rituals that help you unwind? If yes, please describe.

8. **Physical Activity**
- How often do you engage in physical activity?
  - Daily
  - Several times a week
  - Occasionally
  - Never
- What types of physical activity do you enjoy (e.g., walking, yoga, running)?

9. **Stress and Relaxation**
- On a scale of 1-10, how would you rate your current stress levels?
- What are your primary sources of stress?
- What activities or practices help you relax and manage stress?

10. **Daily Schedule**
- Please outline your typical daily schedule, including work, meals, exercise, self-care, and leisure activities.

Analysis And Integration

1. **Identify Opportunities for Herbal Integration**
- Look for times in your daily routine where you can easily incorporate herbal remedies. For example, if you have a morning or evening self-care routine, consider adding an herbal tea to this ritual.

2. **Leverage Preferred Methods**

- Use your preferred methods of herbal consumption to ensure consistency and enjoyment. If you enjoy herbal teas, make them a regular part of your hydration routine. If you prefer capsules, set a reminder to take them.

3. **Combine with Existing Habits**

- Integrate herbal use with existing habits to make it more manageable. For example, if you already drink a lot of water, you might infuse it with herbs like lemon balm or mint. If you have a skincare routine, consider using hydrosols, herb-infused oils or salves.

4. **Adjust and Reflect**

- Regularly assess how well your herbal integration is working. Adjust as needed based on your experiences and any changes in your routine or needs. Reflect on the benefits you observe, such as improved sleep, reduced anxiety, or better overall well-being.

By understanding your daily habits and routines, you can find the best ways to incorporate herbal remedies into your life, ensuring that they become a sustainable and effective part of your sobriety journey.

Confucius

"It does not matter how slowly you go as long as you do not stop."

CHAPTER 2: OVERVIEW OF HERBAL CATEGORIES AND THEIR IMPORTANCE IN SOBRIETY

Before we dive into the detailed chapters on specific herbs and their practical applications, it's important to understand the broader categories of herbs and how they can support your sobriety journey. In this section, we will explore three key categories of herbs: detoxifying herbs, nervine herbs, and adaptogenic herbs. Each category plays a unique role in promoting overall health and well-being, particularly during the process of overcoming alcohol dependence.

Detoxifying Herbs

Detoxifying herbs are essential for cleansing the body and supporting the organs involved in detoxification, such as the liver, kidneys, and lymphatic system. These herbs help to remove toxins that have accumulated due to alcohol consumption and other environmental factors. By promoting efficient detoxification, these herbs aid in restoring balance and vitality to the body.

Key Benefits:

- **Liver Support:** Detoxifying herbs like dandelion and milk thistle help protect and regenerate liver cells, enhancing the liver's ability to filter and eliminate toxins.
- **Kidney Function:** Herbs such as burdock root and nettle act as diuretics, increasing urine production to flush out toxins through the kidneys.
- **Blood Purification:** Burdock root and red clover help cleanse the blood, removing impurities and supporting overall health.

Examples of Detoxifying Herbs:

- Dandelion (Taraxacum officinale)
- Burdock Root (Arctium lappa)
- Milk Thistle (Silybum marianum)
- Nettle (Urtica dioica)
- Red Clover (Trifolium pratense)

Nervine Herbs

Nervine herbs are crucial for managing the emotional and mental challenges associated with sobriety. These herbs have calming and soothing effects on the nervous system, helping to alleviate anxiety, stress, and mood swings. Incorporating nervine herbs into your daily routine can promote relaxation, improve sleep quality, and enhance overall mental well-being.

Key Benefits:

- **Anxiety Relief:** Herbs like chamomile and lemon balm have mild sedative effects, reducing feelings of anxiety and promoting a sense of calm.
- **Stress Reduction:** Nervine herbs such as skullcap

and passionflower help to lower stress levels and support emotional balance.

- **Improved Sleep:** Chamomile and valerian root are particularly effective in promoting restful sleep, which is essential for recovery and overall health.

Examples of Nervine Herbs:

- Chamomile (Matricaria chamomilla)
- Lemon Balm (Melissa officinalis)
- Valerian Root (Valeriana officinalis)
- Passionflower (Passiflora incarnata)
- Skullcap (Scutellaria lateriflora)

Adaptogenic Herbs

Adaptogenic herbs are unique in their ability to help the body adapt to stress and maintain homeostasis. These herbs support the adrenal glands and enhance the body's resilience to physical and emotional stressors. By balancing various physiological processes, adaptogenic herbs contribute to improved energy levels, mental clarity, and overall vitality.

Key Benefits:

- **Stress Resilience:** Adaptogens like ashwagandha and holy basil help the body cope with stress more effectively, reducing the impact of stress on the body and mind.
- **Energy Boost:** Ginseng and rhodiola enhance physical and mental stamina, combating fatigue and improving overall energy levels.
- **Hormonal Balance:** Herbs such as holy basil support hormonal balance, which is crucial for maintaining mood stability and overall health.

Examples of Adaptogenic Herbs:

- Ashwagandha (Withania somnifera)

- Holy Basil (Ocimum sanctum)
- Ginseng (Panax ginseng)
- Rhodiola (Rhodiola rosea)
- Schisandra (Schisandra chinensis)

Importance In The Sobriety Journey

The journey to sobriety involves not only eliminating alcohol from your life but also addressing the physical, emotional, and mental challenges that arise during this process. Detoxifying, nervine, and adaptogenic herbs each play a vital role in supporting different aspects of this journey:

Physical Detoxification: Detoxifying herbs help cleanse the body of toxins, supporting liver and kidney function, and promoting overall physical health. This is a crucial first step in recovery, as it helps the body heal from the damage caused by alcohol.

Emotional and Mental Well-being: Nervine herbs provide essential support for managing anxiety, stress, and mood swings. By promoting relaxation and improving sleep, these herbs help stabilize your emotions and enhance your mental resilience.

Stress Adaptation and Energy: Adaptogenic herbs boost your body's ability to cope with stress, improve energy levels, and maintain hormonal balance. This support is essential for maintaining motivation, focus, and overall vitality during the sobriety journey.

By understanding the unique benefits of these herbal categories and how they can support your sobriety, you can make informed choices about which herbs to incorporate into your routine. In the following chapters, we will dive deeper into each category, exploring specific herbs, their benefits, and practical ways to use them.

Victor Hugo

"Even the darkest night will end and the sun will rise."

DETOXIFYING HERBS

Detoxification is a vital first step in the journey to sobriety. Our bodies accumulate toxins from various sources, including alcohol, processed foods, and environmental pollutants. These toxins can impede our body's natural healing processes, making it harder to achieve and maintain sobriety. Fortunately, nature provides us with powerful allies in the form of detoxifying herbs. These herbs support our liver, kidneys, and lymphatic system, helping to flush out toxins and restore balance.

When we detoxify our bodies, we can experience a wide range of positive changes. As the body sheds accumulated toxins, we often notice increased energy and vitality. Many people report feeling more balanced and centered, both physically and emotionally. Mental clarity can improve significantly, making it easier to focus on personal goals and maintain a positive outlook on life. Detoxification sets the foundation for overall well-being, paving the way for a successful and sustained journey to sobriety.

In this chapter, we will explore some of the most effective detoxifying herbs and how to incorporate them into your daily routine.

Dandelion (Taraxacum Officinale)

Uses: Herbal teas, capsules, tinctures

Benefits: Promotes liver detoxification, acts as a diuretic to flush out toxins

Dandelion is a well-known and widely used herb for liver support and detoxification. Its roots and leaves are rich in vitamins and minerals, including vitamins A, C, and K, as well as calcium and potassium. Dandelion's diuretic properties help the kidneys eliminate waste, while its bitter compounds stimulate liver function and bile production.

Preparation:

- **Herbal Tea:** Steep 1-2 teaspoons of dried dandelion root in a cup of hot water for 10-15 minutes. Strain and drink 1-2 cups daily. Alternatively, try roasting the root before brewing the tea.
- **Tincture:** Use a dandelion root tincture, taking 20-30 drops in a glass of water up to three times a day.
- **Capsules:** Take dandelion root capsules as directed on the product label, usually 500 mg 1-2 times daily.
- **Fresh:** The leaves of the dandelion can be used fresh in salads.

Nettle (Urtica Dioica)

Uses: Herbal teas, capsules, tinctures, fresh

Benefits: Supports kidney function, reduces inflammation, rich in vitamins and minerals

Nettle is a nutrient-dense herb known for its anti-inflammatory and diuretic properties. It supports kidney function by promoting the elimination of waste products and excess fluids. Nettle is rich in vitamins A, C, and K, as well as iron, calcium, and magnesium, making it a valuable addition to any detox regimen.

Preparation:

- **Herbal Tea:** Steep 1-2 teaspoons of dried nettle leaves in a cup of hot water for 10-15 minutes. Strain and drink 1-3 cups daily.

- **Tincture:** Use a nettle tincture, taking 20-30 drops in a glass of water up to three times a day.
- **Capsules:** Take nettle leaf capsules as directed on the product label, usually 300-500 mg 1-2 times daily.
- **Fresh:** Young nettle leaves can be steamed or used in soups and stews. Always handle with gloves to avoid the stinging hairs.

Red Clover (Trifolium Pratense)

Uses: Herbal teas, capsules, tinctures, fresh **Benefits:** Purifies the blood, supports hormonal balance, reduces inflammation

Red clover is traditionally used for its blood-purifying properties and is known to support hormonal balance and reduce inflammation. It contains phytoestrogens, which can help alleviate menopausal symptoms and promote overall hormonal health.

Preparation:

- **Herbal Tea:** Steep 1-2 teaspoons of dried red clover flowers in a cup of hot water for 10-15 minutes. Strain and drink 1-3 cups daily.
- **Tincture:** Use a red clover tincture, taking 20-30 drops in a glass of water up to three times a day.
- **Capsules:** Take red clover capsules as directed on the product label, usually 300-500 mg 1-2 times daily.
- **Fresh:** Red clover flowers can be added to salads or used as a garnish.

Burdock Root (Arctium Lappa)

Uses: Herbal teas, tinctures, capsules

Benefits: Purifies the blood, supports liver function

Burdock root is another excellent herb for detoxification. It has been traditionally used to cleanse the blood and support liver health. Burdock root contains antioxidants like quercetin and luteolin, which help protect the liver from damage and promote the elimination of toxins.Burdock root also contains inulin which helps to improve digestive function.

Preparation:

- **Herbal Tea:** Simmer 1 tablespoon of dried burdock root in 2 cups of water for 20-30 minutes. Strain and drink up to 2 cups daily. Add to a blend like Chai with Ginger, Cardamom and Cinnamon to improve flavor.
- **Tincture:** Take 20-30 drops of burdock root tincture in water up to three times a day.
- **Capsules:** Follow the recommended dosage on the product label, typically 500 mg 1-2 times daily.

Calendula (Calendula Officinalis)

Uses: Herbal teas, tinctures, topical applications
Benefits: Anti-inflammatory, supports lymphatic system, promotes skin health

Calendula is a powerhouse herb renowned for its anti-inflammatory and lymphatic support properties. Internally it helps the body eliminate toxins through the lymphatic system, reducing inflammation and promoting healing.

Additionally, calendula is incredibly beneficial for the skin, which is the body's largest organ and plays a critical role in detoxification. The skin acts as a barrier and a detoxifying organ, eliminating waste through sweat and oil glands. Using calendula externally can support this natural detox process by reducing inflammation, soothing irritated skin, and promoting healing.

Preparation:

- **Herbal Tea:** Steep 1-2 teaspoons of dried calendula flowers in a cup of hot water for 10-15 minutes. Strain and drink 1-2 cups daily.
- **Tincture:** Use calendula tincture, taking 20-30 drops in water up to three times a day. This is the preferred method for internal use
- **Topical Application:** Infuse calendula flowers in oil and apply to the skin to reduce inflammation and promote healing.

Milk Thistle (Silybum Marianum)

Uses: Capsules, tinctures, herbal teas
Benefits: Protects and regenerates liver cells

Milk thistle is one of the most well-known herbs for liver health. It contains silymarin, a compound that has been shown to protect liver cells from toxins and support their regeneration. Milk thistle also has antioxidant and anti-inflammatory properties, making it an essential herb for detoxification.

Preparation:

- **Herbal Tea:** Crush 1 tablespoon of milk thistle seeds and steep in hot water for 10-15 minutes. Strain and drink 1-2 cups daily.
- **Tincture:** Take 20-30 drops of milk thistle tincture in water up to three times a day.
- **Capsules:** Follow the recommended dosage on the product label, typically 200-400 mg of silymarin 1-2 times daily.

How To Incorporate Detoxifying Herbs Into Your Routine

1. **Morning Detox Tea:**
   Start your day with a cup of dandelion or burdock root tea to kickstart your liver's detoxifying processes.
2. **Daily Tinctures:**
   Use tinctures for a quick and convenient way to consume detoxifying herbs. Add them to your water bottle and sip throughout the day.
3. **Herbal Capsules:**
   For those with busy lifestyles, herbal capsules provide an easy way to ensure you're getting your daily dose of detoxifying herbs.
4. **Topical Applications:**
   Use calendula-infused oil or salve to support skin health and reduce inflammation, aiding your body's overall detoxification.
5. **Hydration:**
   Incorporate herbal teas into your hydration routine, replacing or complementing your usual beverages with detoxifying herbal infusions.

Detoxifying your body is a critical step on the path to sobriety. By incorporating these powerful herbs into your daily routine, you can support your body's natural detoxification processes, promote liver health, and pave the way for overall well-being. In the next chapter, we will explore nervine herbs, which are essential for managing anxiety and stress, key challenges in the journey to sobriety.

Helen Keller

"Although the world is full of suffering, it is also full of the overcoming of it."

NERVINE HERBS FOR ANXIETY AND STRESS

The journey to sobriety is often fraught with emotional and mental challenges. Anxiety, stress, and mood swings can make the process of quitting alcohol even more difficult. Nervine herbs, which have calming and soothing effects on the nervous system, can be incredibly beneficial during this time. These herbs help to alleviate anxiety, promote restful sleep, and reduce overall stress levels, allowing you to maintain emotional balance and mental clarity.

Personally, nervine herbs have been instrumental in helping me navigate the outside social world while being alcohol free. Social situations that once triggered anxiety and cravings became more manageable with the support of these calming herbs. They provided a sense of inner peace and stability, allowing me to engage with others more comfortably and confidently without the need for alcohol.

In this chapter, we will explore some of the most effective nervine herbs and how to incorporate them into your daily routine.

American Skullcap (Scutellaria Lateriflora)

Uses: Herbal teas, tinctures, capsules

Benefits: Reduces anxiety, soothes the nervous system

American skullcap is a powerful nervine herb that has been used for centuries to reduce anxiety and calm the nervous system. It contains flavonoids that have a relaxing effect on the body, making it an excellent choice for those dealing with stress and nervous tension. American Skullcap is very useful for acute situations involving panic attacks.

American Skullcap should be avoided by those taking SSRIs.

Preparation:

- **Herbal Tea:** Steep 1-2 teaspoons of dried skullcap in a cup of hot water for 10-15 minutes. Strain and drink 1-2 cups daily.
- **Tincture:** Use a skullcap tincture, taking 20-30 drops in a glass of water up to three times a day.
- **Capsules:** Take skullcap capsules as directed on the product label, usually 300-600 mg 1-2 times daily.

Passionflower (Passiflora Incarnata)

Uses: Herbal teas, tinctures, capsules
Benefits: Eases anxiety, promotes restful sleep

Passionflower is renowned for its ability to ease anxiety and promote restful sleep. It works by increasing levels of gamma-aminobutyric acid (GABA) in the brain, which helps to reduce brain activity and induce a sense of calm.

Passionflower should be avoided by those who are pregnant and/or nursing.

Preparation:

- **Herbal Tea:** Steep 1-2 teaspoons of dried passionflower in a cup of hot water for 10-15 minutes. Strain and drink 1-2 cups daily.
- **Tincture:** Take 20-30 drops of passionflower tincture in

water up to three times a day.

- **Capsules:** Follow the recommended dosage on the product label, typically 300-400 mg 1-2 times daily.

Lemon Balm (Melissa Officinalis)

Uses: Herbal teas, tinctures, capsules
Benefits: Calms the mind, alleviates stress

Lemon balm is a gentle, soothing herb that has been used for centuries to calm the mind and alleviate stress. Its mild sedative properties make it an excellent choice for reducing anxiety and promoting relaxation.

Those with Hypo-thyroidism and/or taking medication for this condition should avoid Lemon Balm.

Preparation:

- **Herbal Tea:** Brew 1-2 teaspoons of dried lemon balm leaves in a cup of hot water for 10-15 minutes. Strain and drink 1-2 cups daily.
- **Tincture:** Use lemon balm tincture, taking 20-30 drops in water up to three times a day.
- **Capsules:** Take lemon balm capsules as directed on the product label, usually 300-500 mg 1-2 times daily.

Chamomile (Matricaria Chamomilla)

Uses: Herbal teas, tinctures
Benefits: Promotes relaxation, soothes digestive issues

Chamomile is one of the most well-known herbs for promoting relaxation and reducing anxiety and tension. Its mild sedative effects help to calm the mind and body, making it easier to unwind and sleep. Chamomile is also beneficial for soothing digestive issues that can be exacerbated by stress.

Preparation:

- **Herbal Tea:** Steep 1-2 teaspoons of dried chamomile flowers in a cup of hot water for 5-10 minutes. Strain and drink 1-2 cups daily.
- **Tincture:** Take 20-30 drops of chamomile tincture in water up to three times a day.

Valerian Root (Valeriana Officinalis)

Uses: Capsules
Benefits: Induces relaxation, helps with sleep

Valerian root is a potent herb for inducing relaxation and promoting deep, restful sleep. It is often used as a natural remedy for insomnia and anxiety. Valerian root works by increasing GABA levels in the brain, similar to passionflower but with a greater sedative effect.

Preparation:

- **Capsules:** Follow the recommended dosage on the product label, typically 300-600 mg an hour before bed. Use for 3 weeks, take 1 week off, then resume.

How To Incorporate Nervine Herbs Into Your Routine

1. **Relaxation Tea:**
   - End your day with a calming cup of chamomile, passionflower and skullcap tea to help you unwind and prepare for a restful night's sleep.
2. **Daily Tinctures:**
   - Use tinctures of skullcap or passionflower for quick and effective relief from anxiety and stress. Add them to your water bottle and sip throughout the day as needed.

3. **Herbal Capsules:**
- For convenience, take valerian root as part of your evening routine to maintain a balanced sleep schedule.

4. **Hydration:**
- Incorporate nervine herbal teas into your hydration routine, replacing or complementing your usual beverages with calming herbal infusions.

Managing anxiety and stress is a crucial aspect of the sobriety journey. By incorporating these powerful nervine herbs into your daily routine, you can support your nervous system, promote relaxation, and maintain emotional balance. In the next chapter, we will explore adaptogenic herbs, which help bring the body into homeostasis and enhance overall resilience to stress.

Buddha

"No matter how hard the past, you can always begin again."

ADAPTOGENIC HERBS FOR BALANCE AND RESILIENCE

Adaptogenic herbs are a special class of plants that help the body adapt to stress, improve resilience, and bring about a state of balance or homeostasis. Unlike other herbs that target specific symptoms or ailments, adaptogens work holistically, supporting multiple body systems to enhance overall health and well-being. These herbs can be particularly beneficial during the sobriety journey, as they help to stabilize mood, boost energy levels, and support the body's ability to cope with physical and emotional stress. In this chapter, we will explore some of the most effective adaptogenic herbs and how to incorporate them into your daily routine.

Holy Basil (Ocimum Sanctum)

Uses: Herbal teas, tinctures, capsules
Benefits: Reduces stress, balances hormones, supports immune function

Holy basil, also known as tulsi, is revered in Ayurvedic medicine for its ability to reduce stress and promote mental clarity. It helps to balance cortisol levels, the body's primary stress hormone, and has powerful antioxidant and anti-inflammatory properties that support overall health.

Preparation:

- **Herbal Tea:** Steep 1-2 teaspoons of dried holy basil leaves in a cup of hot water for 10-15 minutes. Strain and drink 1-2 cups daily.
- **Tincture:** Take 20-30 drops of holy basil tincture in water up to three times a day.
- **Capsules:** Follow the recommended dosage on the product label, typically 300-500 mg 1-2 times daily.

Ashwagandha (Withania Somnifera)

Uses: Capsules, tinctures, herbal teas
Benefits: Supports adrenal health, improves resilience to stress, enhances energy and stamina

Ashwagandha is a well-known adaptogen that has been used for centuries in Ayurvedic medicine. It is highly effective at supporting adrenal health, which can be particularly important during recovery from alcohol dependence. Ashwagandha helps to reduce anxiety, improve sleep, and boost overall energy levels.

Preparation:

- **Herbal Tea:** Add 1 teaspoon of ashwagandha powder to a cup of hot water or milk. Simmer for 10 minutes, then strain and drink.
- **Tincture:** Take 20-30 drops of ashwagandha tincture in water up to three times a day.
- **Capsules:** Follow the recommended dosage on the product label, typically 300-600 mg 1-2 times daily.

Schisandra (Schisandra Chinensis)

Uses: Capsules, tinctures, herbal teas
Benefits: Enhances physical performance, supports liver health, promotes mental clarity

Schisandra is a powerful adaptogen that has been used in Traditional Chinese Medicine for thousands of years. It is known for its ability to enhance physical performance, support liver health, and improve mental clarity. Schisandra berries are rich in antioxidants and help to protect the body from the damaging effects of stress.

Preparation:

- **Herbal Tea:** Simmer 1 tablespoon of dried schisandra berries in 2 cups of water for 20-30 minutes. Strain and drink up to 2 cups daily.
- **Tincture:** Take 20-30 drops of schisandra tincture in water up to three times a day.
- **Capsules:** Follow the recommended dosage on the product label, typically 500-1000 mg 1-2 times daily.

Ginseng (Panax Ginseng)

Uses: Capsules, tinctures, herbal teas
Benefits: Boosts energy, supports overall vitality, enhances cognitive function

Ginseng is one of the most well-known adaptogenic herbs, revered for its ability to boost energy levels, enhance cognitive function, and support overall vitality. Both Asian ginseng (Panax ginseng) and American ginseng (Panax quinquefolius) are effective adaptogens, though they have slightly different properties.

Preparation:

- **Herbal Tea:** Steep 1-2 teaspoons of dried ginseng root in a cup of hot water for 10-15 minutes. Strain and drink 1-2 cups daily.

- **Tincture:** Take 20-30 drops of ginseng tincture in water up to three times a day.
- **Capsules:** Follow the recommended dosage on the product label, typically 200-400 mg 1-2 times daily.

How To Incorporate Adaptogenic Herbs Into Your Routine

Morning Energy Boost:

- Start your day with a cup of holy basil or ginseng tea to boost your energy levels and enhance your resilience to stress.

Daily Tinctures:

- Use tinctures of holy basil or schisandra for a quick and convenient way to support your body's stress response. Add them to your water bottle and sip throughout the day.

Herbal Capsules:

- For those with busy lifestyles, herbal capsules provide an easy way to ensure you're getting your daily dose of adaptogenic herbs.

Evening Relaxation:

- Wind down with a calming cup of ashwagandha turmeric milk in the evening to help reduce stress and promote mental clarity.

Hydration:

- Incorporate adaptogenic herbal teas into your hydration routine, replacing or complementing your usual beverages with balancing herbal infusions.

Adaptogenic herbs are powerful allies in the journey to sobriety.

By incorporating these herbs into your daily routine, you can enhance your body's resilience to stress, boost your energy levels, and maintain a state of balance and well-being. In the next chapter, we will explore various methods of using herbs, including teas, tinctures, capsules, and more, to help you integrate these natural remedies seamlessly into your life.

J.K. Rowling

"Rock bottom became the solid foundation on which I rebuilt my life."

CHAPTER 3: METHODS OF USING HERBS

I ncorporating herbs into your daily routine can be both simple and enjoyable. There are various methods to prepare and use herbs, each offering unique benefits and ways to experience their healing properties. In this chapter, we will explore different methods of using herbs, including herbal teas, tinctures, capsules, herb-infused oils, and hydrosols. Understanding these methods will empower you to choose the best ways to integrate herbs into your lifestyle and support your journey to sobriety.

Herbal Teas

Herbal teas, or tisanes, are one of the simplest and most effective ways to enjoy the benefits of herbs. By steeping herbs in hot water, you can extract their beneficial compounds and create a soothing, therapeutic beverage.

Preparation:

- **Loose Leaf Tea:** Use 1 teaspoon to 1 tablespoon of dried herbs per cup of hot water. Steep for 5-10 minutes, strain, and enjoy.
- **Tea Bags:** Pre-packaged tea bags are convenient and easy

to use. Follow the instructions on the packaging for the best results.

- **Cold Brew:** For a refreshing alternative, cold brew your herbal tea by steeping the herbs in cold water for 6-12 hours. Strain and serve over ice.
- **Sun Tea:** Infuse your herbal concoction with the Suns healing Rays by leaving it outside for several hours.

Benefits:

- **Hydration:** Herbal teas contribute to your daily fluid intake, helping to keep you hydrated.
- **Added Vitamins and Minerals:** Herbs have an array of vitamins, mineral and beneficial plant components that contribute to the body's overall health and function.
- **Customization:** You can mix and match different herbs to create blends that suit your taste and specific health needs.
- **Calming Ritual:** Preparing and drinking herbal tea can be a calming ritual that promotes mindfulness and relaxation.

Tinctures

Tinctures are concentrated herbal extracts made by soaking herbs in a solvent, typically alcohol. They are potent, easy to use, discrete, and have a long shelf life. For those in recovery, tinctures are available that are made with apple cider vinegar or glycerine.

Preparation:

- **Vinegar-Based Tinctures:** Fill a jar ⅓ full with dried herbs or ¾ full of fresh herbs and cover it with apple cider vinegar. Seal the jar with a piece of parchment between the lid and the jar to prevent the vinegar from corroding the metal lid, and let it sit for 4-6 weeks, shaking daily. Once finished, strain the liquid into a dark glass bottle for storage.
- **Glycerin-Based Tinctures:** Use vegetable glycerin as the solvent, following the same preparation steps. Glycerin

tinctures are sweet and alcohol-free, making them ideal for those with alcohol sensitivities.

Benefits:

- **Convenience:** Tinctures are easy to take and can be added to water, tea, or juice.
- **Potency:** Because tinctures are concentrated, you only need a small amount to experience the herb's benefits.
- **Versatility:** Tinctures can be made with a wide variety of herbs, allowing you to create personalized blends.

Capsules And Tablets

Herbal capsules and tablets are a convenient way to consume herbs, especially for those who prefer not to taste the herbs directly. They are available in health food stores or can be made at home using a capsule machine.

Preparation:

- **Store-Bought:** Follow the dosage instructions on the product label.
- **Homemade:** Purchase empty capsules and a capsule machine. Fill the capsules with powdered herbs and seal them according to the machine's instructions.

Benefits:

- **Consistency:** Capsules and tablets provide a consistent dosage, making it easy to manage your herbal intake.
- **Convenience:** They are portable and easy to incorporate into your daily supplement routine.
- **Taste-Free:** Capsules and tablets are ideal for those who dislike the taste of certain herbs.

Herb-Infused Oils

Herb-infused oils are created by steeping herbs in a carrier oil, such as olive oil, coconut oil, avocado oil. or jojoba oil. Different oils can be created for different purposes such as, culinary applications, skincare, and massage. With the skin being the body's largest organ, topical applications of herbs can help with detoxification breakouts, dermatitis, inflammation, acne, eczema and other skin issues you may encounter.

Preparation:

- **Solar Infusion:** Using dried herbs only, fill a jar half way with herbs and cover it with carrier oil. Seal the jar and place it in a sunny spot for 4-6 weeks. Strain the oil into a clean bottle for storage.
- **Heat Infusion:** Combine herbs and oil in a double boiler. Heat gently over very low heat for 1-2 hours, then strain and store the oil.

Benefits:

- **Culinary Uses:** Infused oils can be used in cooking, adding flavor and health benefits to your meals.
- **Skincare:** Apply infused oils directly to the skin to soothe and moisturize. They can also be used as a base for making salves and balms.
- **Massage:** Use infused oils for therapeutic massage to relax muscles and nourish the skin.

Hydrosols

Hydrosols, also known as flower waters, are the aromatic water produced during the steam distillation of plants. They contain water-soluble plant compounds, beneficial acids, microdroplets of essential oils and plant cellular water. These living waters are used both internally and externally, in skincare as facial and body sprays, lotions and serums, in aromatherapy for their olfactory therapeutic purpose, and in culinary applications such as the use of rose water in deserts.

Preparation:

- **Distillation:** A copper alembic still is traditionally used, however a makeshift, stovetop version can also be used. Place fresh herbs in the distiller with water. Assemble the still components and seal. Heat the still to produce steam, which passes through the herbs, travels through a cool, coiled condenser and collects as hydrosol in a separate container.
- **Store-Bought:** Purchase hydrosols from reputable suppliers and use them according to the instructions on the label.

Benefits:

- **Gentle:** Hydrosols are less concentrated than essential oils and very user friendly, making them gentle enough for use on sensitive skin, pets and children.
- **Versatile:** Use hydrosols as facial toners, room sprays, or in cooking and internally adding to your water, tea or coffee.
- **Aromatherapy:** Hydrosols can be used in aromatherapy to promote relaxation and well-being, improve focus and mental clarity and induce relaxation as well as creativity..

How To Choose The Best Method For You

Choosing the best method for incorporating herbs into your routine depends on your personal preferences, lifestyle, and specific health needs. Here are some tips to help you decide:

Consider Your Routine: If you have a busy schedule, capsules and tinctures might be the most convenient options. If you enjoy a daily ritual, herbal teas or infused oils might be more suitable.

Taste Preferences: If you dislike the taste of certain herbs, capsules or tinctures can help you avoid the flavor while still reaping the benefits.

Health Goals: Tailor your herbal use to your specific health goals.

For example, use calming herbal teas for relaxation, or infused oils for skincare and massage.

Experiment: Try different methods and see what works best for you. You might find that a combination of methods suits your needs perfectly.

Incorporating herbs into your daily routine can be a rewarding and effective way to support your health and well-being. By exploring the various methods of using herbs, you can find the best ways to integrate these natural remedies into your lifestyle. In the next chapter, we will delve into my personal journey with herbs, sharing how they have transformed my life and supported my sobriety.

Steve Maraboli

> *"Life doesn't get easier or more forgiving; we get stronger and more resilient."*

CHAPTER 4: 25 HERBAL RECIPES FOR RECOVERY

Incorporating herbs into your daily routine can be both enjoyable and therapeutic. To help you get started, I've compiled 25 herbal recipes that are simple to prepare and effective in supporting your sobriety journey. These recipes include herbal teas, tinctures, salves, and more, each designed to enhance your well-being and support your recovery. Let these recipes inspire you to explore the wonderful world of herbal remedies and experience their incredible benefits.

Detoxifying Teas - These Blends Help Cleanse And Nourish.

1. **Dandelion Detox Tea**

   Ingredients: 1 tsp dried dandelion root, 1 tsp dried or fresh ginger root, 1 tsp dried parsley, slice of lemon, 2 cups water

   Instructions: Simmer roots in water for 20 minutes, adding the parsley and lemon for the last 5 minutes. Strain, sweeten if desired, and enjoy.

2. **Licorice Liver Cleanse**
   Ingredients: 1 tsp dried dandelion, 1 tsp dried burdock, 1 tsp licorice root, 2 cups hot water
   Instructions: Simmer herbs for 15-20 minutes. Strain, sweeten if desired, and enjoy.

3. **Nettle and Red Clover Tea**
   Ingredients: 1 tsp dried nettle leaves, 1 tsp calendula, 1 tsp burdock root, 1 tsp dried red clover flowers, slice of orange peel, 2 cups hot water
   Instructions: Simmer burdock root and calendula on low for 15 minutes. Add red clover, nettles and orange peel in the last 5 minutes.Strain, sweeten if desired, and enjoy.

Calming Teas - These Blends Can Help With Stress, Anxiety And Overwhelm And Help Promote A Sense Of Relaxation, Calm And Balance

4. **Chamomile and Lavender Sleep Tea** - Calm down from the days tension and frustration with this blend.
   Ingredients: 1 tsp dried chamomile flowers, 1/2 tsp dried lavender flowers, 1 cup hot water
   Instructions: Steep herbs in hot water for 5-10 minutes. Strain, sweeten if desired, and enjoy before bedtime to promote a restful sleep.

5. **Wholly Relaxation Tea -** Relaxed and alert.
   Ingredients: 1 tsp dried passionflower, 1 tsp dried lemon balm, 1 tsp dried or fresh holy basil, 2 cups hot water
   Instructions: Steep herbs in hot water for 7-10 minutes. Strain, sweeten if desired, and drink a cup when you are feeling overwhelmed or anxious.

6. **Take it Easy Tea** - Relieve stress, anxiety and overwhelm.

   Ingredients: 1 tsp american skullcap, 1 tsp passionflower, 1 tsp chamomile, 1 cup hot water

   Instructions: Pour hot water over herbs and let steep for 7-10 minutes. Strain and sweeten if desired. Drink when you need to turn down the anxiety, nervousness and tension.

Energizing Teas - Revitalizing Blends That Promote A Calm And Balanced Alertness.

7. **Holy Basil and Ginger Morning Boost** - These 2 herbs are fantastic together and make a perfect wake-me-up blend.

   Ingredients: 1 tsp dried holy basil leaves, 1/2 tsp fresh grated ginger, 1 cup hot water

   Instructions: Steep holy basil and ginger in hot water for 5-10 minutes. Strain, sweeten, and enjoy.

8. **Afternoon Delight** - Great for a midday pick-me-up.

   Ingredients: 1 tsp dried ginseng root, 1 tsp lemongrass, 1 tsp dried peppermint, 1 cup hot water

   Instructions: Steep herbs in hot water for 10-15 minutes. Strain, sweeten if desired, and enjoy.

9. **Schisandra Berry Energy Tea** - A fruity and refreshing tea that is mineral rich and healthy.

   Ingredients: 1 tbsp dried schisandra berries, 1 tsp raspberry leaf, slice of lemon peel, 2 cups water

   Instructions: Simmer schisandra berries in water for 20-30 minutes, strain out the berries and pour the hot liquid over the raspberry leaf & lemon peel, let steep for 5 minutes. Strain and enjoy.

Tinctures: My Top 3 Go-To Tinctures For Detox And Digestion, Stress, Anxiety And The Onset Of A Panic Attack.

10. **O'Dandelion Tincture** - this is a powerful digestive bitters

    Ingredients: Dandelion root, burdock root, organic orange peel, apple cider vinegar

    Instructions: Fill a jar ⅓ full with the roots and orange peel and cover with vinegar. Seal tightly placing a piece of parchment paper between the glass and metal lid to prevent corrosion, and let sit for 6 weeks, shaking daily. Strain well when ready and store in a dark amber bottle making sure to label and date. Take 15 minutes before eating to stimulate digestive fluids and aid in healthy digestion.

11. **Holy Basil Tincture** - I refer to this as, "my energetic coat of armor".

    Ingredients: Holy basil leaves,fresh or dried, apple cider vinegar.

    Instructions: Fill a jar with fresh leaves or ¾ full of dried and cover with vinegar or glycerine. Seal and let sit for 4-6 weeks, shaking daily. Strain and store in a dark bottle making sure to properly label and date.

12. **American Skullcap Tincture** - For acute situations of stress, anxiety, panic and overwhelm. I always take this with me when I leave the house. I make a blend of skullcap, passionflower, chamomile and rose petals.

    Ingredients: American skullcap herb, apple cider vinegar or glycerine.

    Instructions: Fill a jar ¾ full with dried skullcap and cover with vinegar. Seal well placing a piece of parchment between the glass and the metal lid to prevent corrosion. Let it sit for 4-6 weeks, shaking daily. Strain and store in a dark bottle making sure to label and date.

Capsules - Easy To Find And Convenient, Capsules Are A Great Alternative To Teas And Tinctures.

13. **Ashwagandha Capsules** - An adaptogen useful for maintaining hormone balance and homeostasis in the body.
    Ingredients: Ashwagandha powder, empty capsules
    Instructions: Use a capsule machine to fill empty capsules with ashwagandha powder. Daily recommended dosage is between 250-600 mg for at least 8 weeks.

14. **Serenity Slumber Capsules** - Useful for acute panic and anxiety attacks, and sleep issues.
    Ingredients: American Skullcap, Passionflower, Hops, Valerian root powders, empty capsules
    Instructions: Use a capsule machine to fill empty capsules with equal parts of each powder. Dosage is 1-2 capsules, depending on body weight, an hour before sleep.

15. **Valerian Root Capsules** - A powerful sleep aid.
    Ingredients: Valerian root powder, empty capsules
    Instructions: Use a capsule machine to fill empty capsules with valerian root powder. Take 1-2 capsules, depending on weight, an hour before sleep.

Infused Oils - Easy To Make And Chemical Free, Herb Infused Oils Have Replaced

All Of My Otc Lotions And Potions.

16. **Calendula Infused Oil** - A very useful oil to always have on hand for external use of dermatitis, inflammation, dry, itchy skin, wounds, eczema and more.
    Ingredients: Dried calendula flowers, olive oil
    Instructions: Fill a jar with dried calendula flowers and cover with olive oil. Seal and place in a sunny spot for 6-8 weeks. Strain and store in a clean bottle.

17. **Chamomile, Lavender and Rose-Infused Face Oil** - Jojoba matches our skin's sebum the most, and so I like it for face oils .
    Ingredients: Dried chamomile, lavender and rose petals, jojoba oil.
    Instructions: Fill a jar with the dried flowers and cover with jojoba oil. Seal and place in a sunny spot for 4-6 weeks. Strain and store in a clean bottle.

18. **Sore Muscle Massage Oil-Infused Oil** - Use this massage oil as a part of your ongoing self care routine. It deeply penetrates to release tense muscles and improve blood flow.
    Ingredients: Dried ginger, dried comfrey leaf or root, calendula, lavender, avocado oil
    Instructions: Fill a jar half full with equal parts of each herb and cover with avocado oil. Seal and place in a sunny spot for 6-8 weeks. Strain and store in a clean bottle.

Salves And Balms - Beneficial To Have On Hand For A Variety Of External Uses.

19. **Calendula Healing Salve** - The one must have in my herbal first aid kit, calendula salve is useful for

external dermatitis, cuts and wounds, acne, redness and inflammation, infections, burns, boils, bites and stings and more.

Ingredients: 1 cup calendula-infused oil, 1/4 cup beeswax, ⅛ cup Cocoa Butter

Instructions: Melt beeswax, and cocoa butter in a double boiler. Add the calendula-infused oil and stir until everything is thoroughly dissolved. Remove from heat, and pour into jars. Allow to cool and solidify completely before capping.

20. **Chamomile, Lavender & Rose Sleep Balm** - A wonderful sleep balm, use this for a self massage before bed. .

Ingredients: 1 cup infused oil, 1/4 cup beeswax, ⅛ cup of mango butter, 10 drops lavender essential oil

Instructions: Melt beeswax in a double boiler. Add infused oil and stir until combined. Remove from heat, add lavender essential oil, and pour into jars. Allow to cool and solidify completely before capping.

21. **Peppermint Muscle Relief Balm** - not only is this a cool, tension relieving massage balm, it also makes a fantastic foot balm. Use this and stimulate acupressure points on the foot for stress relief, general selfcare and relaxation.

Ingredients: 1 cup peppermint-infused oil, 1/4 cup beeswax, 10 drops peppermint essential oil

Instructions: Melt beeswax in a double boiler. Add peppermint-infused oil and stir until combined. Remove from heat, add peppermint essential oil, and pour

Smoothies And Herbal Beverages

22. **Ashwagandha Smoothie Boost** - A delicious, adaptogenic beverage any time of the day.
    Ingredients: 1 tsp ashwagandha powder, 1 banana, 1.5 cups almond milk, 1 tbsp honey
    Instructions: Blend all ingredients until smooth. Enjoy as a nutritious and energizing drink.

23. **Ginger Golden Milk** - A warm and soothing drink to ease inflammation and digestive complaints.
    Ingredients: 1 tsp fresh grated ginger, 1 tsp turmeric powder, 3 green cardamom pods, 1 star anise, 1 cinnamon stick, 2 cups of milk, 1 tbsp honey, a pinch of black pepper
    Instructions: Heat all ingredients, except the honey, gently over medium-low heat for 20 minutes, being careful not to boil the milk. Strain into a mug and sweeten with honey. Enjoy as an evening anti-inflammatory beverage.

24. **Green Superfood Smoothie** - Protein, fiber and gut healthy herbs to start the day.
    Ingredients: 1 cup spinach, 1/2 cup kale, 1 banana, 1 cup green tea, 1 tsp burdock root powder, 1 tsp slippery elm, 1 tsp psyllium husks, 1 tsp chlorella powder
    Instructions: Blend all ingredients until smooth. Enjoy as a nutrient-packed, mid day drink.

25. **Rehydrating Herbal Lemonade** - I like making sun tea first then turning it into this refreshing, mineral rich lemonade. Add dried butterfly pea flower for its nootropic benefits and turn it purple!
    Ingredients: 1 quart water, 1/4 cup fresh lemon juice, 1/4 cup honey, 1 tbsp dried nettle leaves, 1 tbsp dried red raspberry leaves
    Instructions: Steep herbs in hot water for 15 minutes

or make a sun tea like me, then strain. Mix the herbal infusion with lemon juice and honey, and chill. Serve over ice for a refreshing and rehydrating drink.

These 25 herbal recipes are just the beginning of what you can make using herbs. Each recipe is designed to support recovery and enhance overall well-being. Experiment with these recipes, find what works best for you, and enjoy the journey of discovering how herbs can transform your life. Remember, the key to success is consistency, so make these herbal practices a regular part of your daily routine. In the next chapter, we will conclude with some final thoughts and encouragement for your ongoing journey to sobriety and health.

Rumi

"The wound is the place where the Light enters you."

CHAPTER 5: TOOLS AND SUPPLIES FOR HERBAL PREPARATIONS

For those wanting to embark on a DIY journey and make their own herbal preparations, some basic tools and supplies are required to prepare and store your herbal remedies effectively. Having the right equipment can make the process easier, more enjoyable, and ensure the highest quality of your herbal products. In this section, we'll go over the essential tools and supplies you'll need for making herbal teas, tinctures, capsules, infused oils, and more.

Basic Tools

Mortar and Pestle

- Used for grinding and crushing herbs into powders or pastes. This traditional tool is ideal for small batches and provides a hands-on way to prepare herbs.

Herb Grinder

- An electric or manual grinder can be used to grind dried herbs quickly and efficiently, especially useful for making teas or powders for capsules..

Measuring Spoons and Cups

- Use these for measuring herbs and liquids by volume.

Strainers and Cheesecloth

- Fine mesh strainers or cheesecloth are used to strain out plant material from liquids when making teas, tinctures, and infusions.

Mason Jars and Glass Containers

- These are essential for storing dried herbs, tinctures, infusions, and other herbal preparations. Glass is preferred because it doesn't react with the herbs and preserves their quality.

Double Boiler

- Useful for making herb-infused oils and salves, a double boiler helps to gently heat herbs without burning them.

Funnel

- A funnel is handy for transferring liquids into bottles or jars without spilling.

Dropper Bottles

- These small glass bottles with droppers are perfect for storing and dispensing tinctures.

Capsule Machine

- If you prefer taking herbs in capsule form, a capsule machine can help you fill empty capsules with herbal powders quickly and efficiently.

Supplies

Dried Herbs

- Purchase high-quality, organic dried herbs from reputable suppliers. Keep a variety of commonly used herbs on hand for different preparations.

Solvents

- **Apple Cider Vinegar:** A non-alcoholic alternative for tinctures.
- **Glycerin:** Another non-alcoholic solvent, often used for making sweet-tasting tinctures for children.

Carrier Oils

- **Olive Oil:** Commonly used for making herb-infused oils.
- **Coconut Oil:** Great for skin preparations due to its solid state at room temperature.
- **Avocado Oil:** Another great option. Check for any known allergies.
- **Jojoba Oil:** A long-lasting oil that closely resembles the skin's natural sebum.

Beeswax & Butters

- Butters such as Cocoa, Shea & Mango, along with Bees Wax are commonly used in making salves and balms to give them a firm texture and add emollience.

Empty Capsules

- Available in various sizes, empty capsules are filled with powdered herbs using a capsule machine.

Labels and Markers

- Label all your herbal preparations with the name of

the herb, date of preparation, and any important usage instructions.

Spray Bottles

- Useful for making herbal sprays and mists, such as hydrosols or room fresheners.

Storage Containers

- Airtight containers for storing your dried herbs and finished products to keep them fresh and potent.

Optional Tools And Supplies

Dehydrator

- If you grow your own herbs, a dehydrator can be very useful for drying them quickly and efficiently.

Herbal Press

- A press can help extract more liquid from your herbal mixtures, making your tinctures and infusions more potent.

Coffee Grinder

- Useful for grinding small quantities of dried herbs into fine powders.

Pipettes

- For accurately measuring small amounts of liquid, especially useful when making tinctures or essential oil blends.

By equipping yourself with these tools and supplies, you will be well-prepared to create a variety of herbal preparations at home. Whether you're making a simple cup of herbal tea or crafting a complex tincture, having the right equipment can make the process smoother and more enjoyable. As you gain experience, you may find additional tools and supplies that enhance your herbal practice, but these basics will provide a strong foundation for your journey into herbal medicine.

CHAPTER 6: KEEP A HERBAL JOURNAL

Keeping a herbal journal is an excellent way to document your journey with herbs, track your progress, and reflect on the changes you experience. This activity encourages mindfulness and self-awareness, helping you to connect more deeply with your herbal allies and their effects on your overall well-being. In this chapter, I'll guide you through the process of starting and maintaining a herbal journal, offering tips, prompts, and insights to make your journaling practice meaningful and beneficial.

Start A Dedicated Herbal Journal

Choosing a Journal

- First, select a notebook or journal specifically for this purpose. It can be as simple or as elaborate as you like. Some may prefer a plain notebook, while others might enjoy a journal with prompts or an herbal theme.

Setting Up Your Journal

Title Page: Start with a title page that includes your

name and the date you started your journal.

Introduction: Write a brief introduction about your goals for using herbs and what you hope to achieve with this journal.

Daily Or Weekly Entries

Date: Begin each entry with the date.

Herbs Used: List the herbs you used that day or week, including the form: tea, tincture, capsule, and dosage.

Preparation Method: Describe how you prepared the herbs. For example, "Steeped 1 teaspoon of chamomile flowers in hot water for 10 minutes."

Time of Day: Note the time of day you used the herbs. This can help identify patterns in how the herbs affect you at different times.

Reason for Use: Explain why you chose these particular herbs. Was it to reduce anxiety, improve sleep, support detoxification, or another reason?

Reflection And Effects

Initial Feelings: Before using the herbs, take a moment to reflect on how you feel. Are you feeling anxious, tired, energized, or something else?

Post-Use Reflections: After using the herbs, note any immediate effects you experience. Did you feel calmer, more alert, less anxious?

Long-Term Effects: At the end of the week or month, reflect on any long-term changes you've noticed. Are you sleeping better? Do you feel more balanced and less stressed?

Herbal Combinations And Blends

Documenting Blends: Document any herbal combinations or blends you create. Note the ingredients, proportions, and why you chose to combine these particular herbs.

Effectiveness of Blends: Reflect on the effectiveness of the blends. Did the combination enhance the effects of the individual herbs?

Symptoms And Improvements

Tracking Symptoms: Track any symptoms you are trying to manage with herbs, such as anxiety, insomnia, digestive issues, or cravings.

Noting Improvements: Note any improvements or changes in these symptoms over time. This can help you determine which herbs are most effective for your needs.

Challenges And Adjustments

Documenting Challenges: Document any challenges you encounter in your herbal practice. This could include issues with consistency, difficulty in preparation, or herbs that didn't seem to work as expected.

Adjusting Practices: Reflect on how you addressed these challenges. Did you adjust dosages, try a different preparation method, or switch to a different herb?

New Discoveries

Exploring New Herbs: Write about any new herbs you try and your experiences with them. Include details about why you decided to try them and what effects you noticed.

Comparing Effects: Reflect on how these new herbs compare to the ones you've been using regularly.

Overall Reflections

Monthly Summaries: At the end of each month, write a summary of your overall experience. Reflect on the progress you've made, any setbacks, and your plans moving forward.

Integrating Practices: Consider how your herbal practices have integrated into your daily life and sobriety journey.

Reflection Prompts

- How did you feel before and after using the herb?
- Did you notice any changes in your mood, energy levels, or overall health?
- What was your experience preparing and using the herb?
- Which herbs have you found to be most effective for your needs?
- Have you encountered any challenges or obstacles in your herbal practice? How did you overcome them?
- What new insights have you gained about your health and well-being through this process?

Benefits Of Keeping A Herbal Journal

Increased Awareness: Regular journaling helps you become more aware of how herbs affect your body and mind, allowing you to make more informed decisions about your herbal practices.

Track Progress: A journal provides a record of your journey, showing how your use of herbs evolves and the benefits you experience over time.

Personalized Insights: By documenting your experiences, you can identify which herbs and methods work best for you, creating a personalized approach to herbal healing.

Motivation and Encouragement: Reflecting on positive changes and progress can motivate you to continue your herbal practices and stay committed to your sobriety journey.

Mindfulness and Reflection: The act of journaling itself can be a mindful practice, encouraging you to reflect on your experiences and connect more deeply with your healing process.

I encourage you to make journaling a regular part of your herbal practice. Use it as a tool for self-discovery, growth, and healing. By keeping a detailed and reflective herbal journal, you can gain valuable insights into your journey and enhance your overall well-being.

Thich Nhat Hanh

"Smile, breathe, and go slowly."

CHAPTER 7: USING TEA RITUALS WITH GUIDED MEDITATION

Incorporating tea rituals with guided meditation into your daily routine can offer profound benefits for relaxing and regulating the nervous system. This practice has been a cornerstone of my personal journey to sobriety and well-being. Something as simple as sitting for 20 minutes in the quiet with a cup of aromatic tea, while listening to crystal bowls, whale sounds, or even gospel music, can do amazing things for the body and mind if you make it a habit. In this chapter, I'll share how you can create your own tea rituals and guided meditations, and how these practices can support your overall health and sobriety.

The Power Of Tea Rituals

Tea rituals are more than just drinking a cup of tea; they are about creating a mindful, intentional experience that engages all your senses. The aroma of the tea, the warmth of the cup, the soothing taste, and the act of slowing down to enjoy the moment has a calming effect on the mind and body. Regularly practicing tea rituals can help reduce stress, improve focus, and promote a sense of peace and well-being.

How To Create Your Own Tea Ritual

Choose Your Tea

Select a tea that aligns with your needs and preferences. For relaxation, consider calming herbs like chamomile or lemon balm. For energy and focus, try green tea, peppermint, or holy basil.

Prepare Your Space

Find a quiet, comfortable place where you can sit undisturbed for your tea ritual. You might want to create a cozy corner with soft cushions, a blanket, and dim lighting.

Set Your Intention

Before you begin, take a moment to set an intention for your tea ritual. This could be something like "I am taking this time to relax and nourish my body and mind" or "I am creating space for peace and clarity."

Brew Your Tea

Prepare your tea mindfully, paying attention to the process. Measure the herbs, boil the water, and steep the tea with care. Let the act of making tea be a meditative experience in itself.

Engage Your Senses

As you drink your tea, engage all your senses. Notice the color of the tea, inhale its aroma, feel the warmth of the cup in your hands, and savor each sip. Allow yourself to be fully present in the moment.

Incorporating Guided Meditation

Adding guided meditation to your tea ritual can deepen the benefits and help you achieve a greater sense of relaxation and balance. Here's how you can incorporate guided meditation into your tea ritual:

Choose Your Meditation

Select a guided meditation that resonates with you. You can find meditations that focus on relaxation, healing, mindfulness, or any theme that supports your current needs. I like journey meditations where I am guided to a secret room that has new opportunities that are awaiting to be discovered. There are many apps and online resources with guided meditations to choose from.

Set Up Your Soundscape

Perhaps you would rather listen to soundscapes or inspiring music.This could be crystal bowls, whale sounds, gospel music, handpan drum, chanting monks, native american flute, or any other calming audio that helps you relax. You can play these sounds softly in the background.

Silence is Golden

Maybe you just sit and listen to the sounds around you, observing your surroundings. Is it raining? Are there cars close by? Do you hear birds or cicadas? If you're really lucky, you get to listen to the silence of the deep forest.

Listen and Sip

Begin your guided meditation or whichever way you choose, and listen attentively as you slowly sip your tea. Allowing the combination of the calming tea and the mindfulness to bring you into a state of deep relaxation.

Reflect and Close

After your time spent in this space, take a few moments to reflect on your experience. Notice how you feel physically, mentally, and emotionally. Close your ritual by expressing gratitude for this time of self-care.

Taking time out for tea and guided meditation became invaluable tools for managing my stress and finding inner peace. I leaned on these practices heavily, especially during challenging times like when I was bored. Sitting quietly with a cup of tea, just being, allowed me to slow down, reconnect with myself and find calm amidst the chaos.

The regular practice of tea rituals and meditation helped me regulate my nervous system, reducing anxiety and promoting a sense of strength of balance. Over time, these teatime rituals became a cherished part of my daily routine, offering a sanctuary of peace and clarity. Making a habit of these practices can provide profound benefits for both the body and mind, supporting your journey to sobriety and overall well-being.

Tips For Making Tea Rituals A Habit

Schedule Your Rituals

Set a specific time each day for your tea ritual and meditation. Consistency is key to making it a habit.

Create Space

Dedicate a specific area in your home, inside or out, for your teatime rituals. Create a mental and energetic space by setting an intention. Having a designated space can help signal to your mind and body that it's time to relax and unwind.

Use Reminders

Set reminders on your phone or create visual cues in your environment to help you remember that it's time for your tea ritual.

Incorporating tea rituals with guided meditation into your daily routine can offer deep benefits for relaxing and regulating the nervous system. These practices can help you find peace, balance, and clarity on your journey to sobriety. By making a habit of these rituals, you can create a sanctuary of calm and well-being in your everyday life. Take the time to explore and enjoy the profound benefits that this time can bring.

Louise Hay

"I am in the process of becoming the best version of myself."

CHAPTER 8: SAFETY AND PRECAUTIONS

When using herbs to support your sobriety journey, it's essential to approach their use with care and awareness. While herbs can offer significant benefits, they can also interact with medications, cause allergic reactions, or have other side effects if not used correctly. This section provides important safety considerations and precautions to ensure you use herbs effectively and safely.

Consulting Healthcare Professionals

1. Seek Professional Advice:
   Always consult with a healthcare professional, such as a doctor or a licensed herbalist, before starting any new herbal regimen. This is especially important if you are currently taking medications or have existing health conditions.
2. Medication Interactions:
   Some herbs can interact with prescription medications, potentially altering their effectiveness or causing adverse effects. A healthcare professional can help you identify any potential interactions and adjust your regimen accordingly.

Allergies And Sensitivities

Identify Allergies:

Before using any new herb, be aware of any known allergies or sensitivities you might have. Perform a patch test when using a new topical herbal preparation to check for any adverse skin reactions.

Start Slowly:

Introduce new herbs gradually, starting with small doses to monitor how your body reacts. If you experience any adverse reactions, discontinue use immediately and consult a healthcare professional.

Dosage And Preparation

Follow Recommended Dosages:

Use herbs in the recommended dosages and avoid exceeding the suggested amounts. More is not always better, and excessive use of some herbs can lead to adverse effects.

Use High-Quality Herbs:

Ensure that you are using high-quality, organic herbs from reputable sources. Contaminated or poor-quality herbs can be ineffective or harmful.

Proper Preparation:

Follow proper preparation methods for herbal teas, tinctures, capsules, and other preparations. Incorrect preparation can reduce the effectiveness of the herbs or introduce harmful substances.

Special Populations

Pregnant or Breastfeeding Women:

> Many herbs are not safe for use during pregnancy or breastfeeding. Always consult with a healthcare professional before using any herbs if you are pregnant or breastfeeding.

Children:

> Herbs can affect children differently than adults. Consult a pediatrician or a licensed herbalist before giving any herbal remedies to children.

Monitoring And Adjusting

Monitor Your Response:

> Keep track of how your body responds to different herbs. Use a herbal journal to note any changes in your symptoms, mood, or overall well-being.

Adjust as Needed:

> Based on your observations and feedback from healthcare professionals, adjust your herbal regimen as needed. It's important to remain flexible and responsive to your body's needs.

Legal Considerations

Regulations and Legality:

> Be aware of the legal status of certain herbs in your country or region. While the herbs in this book are generally regarded as safe, other herbs you may explore

may be regulated or restricted due to their potent effects.

Purchasing and Using Herbs:

Ensure you are purchasing herbs from reputable suppliers who comply with local regulations and quality standards.

Safe Storage

Proper Storage:

Store herbs in a cool, dry place away from direct sunlight to maintain their potency and prevent spoilage.

Labeling:

Clearly label all your herbal preparations with the name of the herb, date of preparation, and any important usage instructions.

By following these safety considerations and precautions, you can use herbs effectively and safely to support your sobriety journey. Remember that while herbs can offer powerful benefits, they must be used with care and respect. Always prioritize your health and well-being by seeking professional guidance and being mindful of how your body responds to these natural remedies. With a thoughtful and informed approach, you can harness the healing power of herbs to enhance your path to sobriety and overall wellness.

Martin Luther King Jr.

"If you can't fly then run, if you can't run then walk, if you can't walk then crawl, but whatever you do you have to keep moving forward."

SUMMARY

The journey to sobriety is a deeply personal and transformative process, and incorporating the healing power of herbs can provide profound support along the way. In this book, we've explored various herbs that can aid in detoxification, calm the mind, and bring the body into balance. We've also delved into practical ways to integrate these herbs into your daily life through teas, tinctures, capsules, and more.

We began with an overview of detoxifying herbs like dandelion, burdock root, and milk thistle, which help cleanse the body and support liver function. We then moved on to nervine herbs such as chamomile, lemon balm, and valerian root, which are essential for managing anxiety and stress. Adaptogenic herbs like holy basil, ashwagandha, and ginseng were also highlighted for their ability to enhance resilience and maintain homeostasis.

Additionally, we discussed the importance of creating herbal rituals, like tea rituals combined with guided meditation, to deepen the benefits and promote overall well-being. Through personal stories and practical advice, we aimed to inspire and empower you to take control of your health using the natural wisdom of herbs.

CONCLUSION

As you continue on your journey to sobriety, remember that healing is a holistic process that involves nurturing your body, mind, and spirit. Herbs can be powerful allies in this journey, offering natural support and enhancing your resilience to stress. By incorporating herbal practices into your daily routine, you can create a foundation of health and well-being that supports your sobriety and enriches your life.

Reflect on the knowledge and tools shared in this book, and feel empowered to experiment with different herbs and methods to find what works best for you. Keep a herbal journal to track your progress and insights, and don't hesitate to seek guidance from healthcare professionals and experienced herbalists as needed.

Your journey is unique, and every step you take towards healing and balance is a victory. Embrace the process, be patient with yourself, and celebrate the progress you make. You have the power to transform your life, and the wisdom of herbs can be a valuable part of that transformation.

Continuing Your Journey

As you move forward, here are some guidelines to help you continue applying the strategies and principles you've learned:

Consistency is Key

Make herbal practices a regular part of your daily routine. Consistency will help you fully experience the benefits of these natural remedies.

Stay Curious and Open

Continue exploring new herbs and methods. Herbalism is a vast field with endless possibilities for discovery and healing.

Listen to Your Body

Pay attention to how your body responds to different herbs and adjust your practices accordingly. Your body's feedback is invaluable in guiding your herbal journey.

Keep a Herbal Journal

Maintain your herbal journal to track your progress, reflect on your experiences, and document any new insights. This practice will help you stay mindful and connected to your healing process.

Seek Support and Community

Don't hesitate to seek guidance from healthcare professionals, herbalists, and supportive communities. Sharing your journey with others can provide additional support and inspiration.

Embrace Mindfulness and Rituals

Incorporate mindfulness practices and rituals into your daily life. Simple rituals like tea meditation can provide a sanctuary of peace and clarity amidst the challenges of daily life.

Celebrate Your Progress

Acknowledge and celebrate your achievements, no matter how small. Every step forward is a testament to your strength and commitment.

FINAL THOUGHTS

Your journey to sobriety and well-being is unique, and embracing the natural support of herbs can enhance and enrich this journey. By integrating the knowledge and practices shared in this book, you are taking proactive steps towards a healthier, more balanced life. Remember, healing is a holistic process that involves nurturing your body, mind, and spirit. Be patient and compassionate with yourself as you continue to grow and transform.

Thank you for allowing me to be a part of your journey. May the wisdom of herbs guide and support you, bringing you peace, health, and fulfillment. Keep moving forward with courage and resilience, and trust in the power of nature to heal and sustain you.

All the Best,

Deidra

HERBAL GLOSSARY

Dandelion (Taraxacum officinale): Promotes liver detoxification, acts as a diuretic to flush out toxins.

Burdock Root (Arctium lappa): Purifies the blood, supports liver function.

Milk Thistle (Silybum marianum): Protects and regenerates liver cells.

Chamomile (Matricaria chamomilla): Promotes relaxation, soothes digestive issues.

Lemon Balm (Melissa officinalis): Calms the mind, alleviates stress.

Valerian Root (Valeriana officinalis): Induces relaxation, helps with sleep.

Holy Basil (Ocimum sanctum): Reduces stress, balances hormones, supports immune function.

Ashwagandha (Withania somnifera): Supports adrenal health, improves resilience to stress, enhances energy and stamina.

Ginseng (Panax ginseng): Boosts energy, supports overall vitality, enhances cognitive function.

This concludes our journey through the healing power of herbs. Remember, your path to sobriety and wellness is unique, and with the support of these natural allies, you can achieve a life of balance, health, and fulfillment.

RESOURCES FOR FURTHER LEARNING

- ❖ Books:
  - ➤ "The Herbal Medicine-Maker's Handbook" by James Green
  - ➤ "Rosemary Gladstar's Medicinal Herbs: A Beginner's Guide" by Rosemary Gladstar
  - ➤ "Adaptogens: Herbs for Strength, Stamina, and Stress Relief" by David Winston
  - ➤ :"The Encyclopedia of Herbal Medicine" by Andrew Chevallier
- ❖ Websites:
  - ➤ American Herbalists Guild
  - ➤ Mountain Rose Herbs Blog
  - ➤ IIerbMentor
- ❖ Courses:
  - ➤ Online courses offered by the Herbal Academy, Evolutionary Herbalism, Herbalista and Chestnut Herbs
  - ➤ Workshops and classes at your local herbalist or health food store
  - ➤ Community college or university courses in herbalism and natural health

ABOUT THE AUTHOR

Deidra is a dedicated backyard herbalist and advocate for holistic health, with a personal journey that has transformed her life. Since overcoming alcohol dependence with the help of herbal allies, she has devoted herself to sharing this wisdom with others.

Deidra offers courses in beginners herbalism and cultivates a large medicinal and botanical beverage garden, creating natural remedies and inspiring others to explore the benefits of herbal medicine. Through her writing and teaching, she aims to empower others to take control of their health and well-being using the natural gifts of the earth.

Contact Information

I would love to hear from you! Whether you have questions, feedback, or stories about your own journey with herbs and sobriety, please feel free to reach out. deidra@highmoonfarm.com

Website: www.highmoonfarm.com

Social Media:

 Instagram: instagram.com/highmoonhomegrownhandmade

Patreon: patreon.com/highmoonfarm

Feel free to reach out with any questions, comments, or to share your experiences. Your journey is important, and I'm here to support you every step of the way.

ACKNOWLEDGMENTS

I would like to express my deepest gratitude to everyone who has supported and inspired me throughout this journey. To my mentors over the years, whose wisdom and guidance have been invaluable. And to all the readers, thank you for embarking on this journey with me. May the knowledge and practices shared in this book bring you healing, peace, and empowerment.

BOOKS IN THIS SERIES

Thriving in Sobriety

I created this series based on the things I did to achieve a life free from alcohol. May these books be a resourse for you on your journey.

Thriving In Sobriety: 25 Fun Ways To Stay Engaged And Inspired

Thriving In Sobriety: 25 More Fun Ways To Stay Engaged And Inspired

9 798333 839114